To my Wife Dorene

Medical Crisis

What Every Caregiver Should Know
Diagnosis, Surgery,
Hospital Stay, Recovery

Peter G. Christie

To order additional copies of this book, contact:
Xlibris Corporation
1-888-795-4274
www.Xlibris.com
Orders@Xlibris.com
86487

CONTENTS

Preface

When someone gets sick, it affects those around them. The reason that I am writing this book is to give those closest to the sick person some things to think about that might be very helpful to both you and your sick relation. Whether you are a spouse, sibling, parent, child, good friend or more distant relative, the more prepared you are now, the more your loved one will benefit in the long run.

All of my opinions and observations are based upon my own personal experience in dealing with my wife's diagnosis, hospital stay and recovery. I think that many people will have a tendency to say, "Yeah, but we're different," or "Yeah, but our hospitals and doctors are better" or any other "Yeah but . . ." you can conjure up.

The truth is that my wife and I may be a bit different than you and your loved one. And, you may be at a better hospital and will be dealing with different medical personnel. However, the commonalities will be very similar.

As you read these passages, try to identify with those that make sense to you and, at the very least, don't judge them but remain open to the possibility that you may have similar experiences. In so doing, you will be better prepared to help your loved one.

By way of background, we are both a young fifty nine years old. By that, I mean that we are more active than most people our age. My wife has worked out in some way, shape or fashion about six days per week for the past 25 years. I am less active and disciplined but still manage to work out about four or five times a week for the past fifteen years.

We are both professional. Her job is an 8:00 am to 4:00 pm in an office setting. She works hard but has relatively little stress in the workplace. My job involves a bit more of a time commitment and although it is primarily a day job, I also have many evening functions.

We were married very young in life, at age 19. We are the proud parents of two sons who are successful, grown, young men and we are the proud grandparents of four grandchildren. We live in the greater Boston area less than a half a mile away from three grandsons and a son and daughter in law. My other son and granddaughter live in Las Vegas.

Our incomes would probably put us in upper middle class. We have little debt and ample savings to provide for us during retirement. We both enjoy doing what we do. My guess is that my wife will work for a few more years and that I will work for a few more after her.

We have both been blessed with health and have had no extreme tragedies in our families. Her parents and siblings are all living. I lost my father 10 years ago but everyone else is doing fine. My wife comes from an Italian family where the kids are all close and everybody knows everybody else's business. My family is Irish and everybody keeps pretty much to themselves.

Both of our parents were hard working. Her father was an entrepreneur. Her mother raised six children. My father was a blue collar worker who made his way to middle management and my mother was a stayed at home Mom who reared the four children in our family. My wife's father was college educated and mine was not. They both put the needs of the family before the needs of themselves.

My wife and I enjoy our family above all other things. We are proud of our sons, love our grandchildren and daughter in law, and are at our happiest when we are all together.

In short, we are pretty normal, non-extravagant people who have worked hard, been careful with our money, and are pretty comfortable in life. The grandchildren are all that any older person has ever said they would be. Our life is, or I should say was, nearly perfect.

All of that changed one day in February of 2010. The day started out about as routine as any. I got up early to get ready for work and hit the shower first. My wife got up after I had dressed and gone done stairs. I don't really remember if we had much to say to one another that morning other than to make a comment or two about the stories on the local news.

I may have heard her say that she was going to a doctor's appointment or I may not have. My wife has allergies so the doctor's office is not uncommon. Plus, she had been having a woman's problem for the past couple of weeks that had come and gone, something about a urinary tract infection.

At any rate, she was bit later than usual getting dressed as was I because I had a meeting in a town nearby and didn't have my norm al 20 mile commute to work. I said good bye and went to my meeting.

As coincidence will have it, or maybe it wasn't a coincidence at all, my meeting ended around 11:00 am and I headed home to get some papers that I had forgotten as I wanted to go to work at my office for the remainder of the day.

As I entered my kitchen, my wife was standing with her back turned to me. I had forgotten about her doctor's appointment. I asked her, "What are you doing home?"

With that, she turned an with a contorted face that I had never before seen, a face that was filled with sorry and fear, she broke down crying and said that words that will change our lives forever: "I've got Cancer!"

Chapter One

"I've Got Cancer"

I returned home unexpectedly from a meeting around 11:30 am one cold winter morning to pick up some papers that I had left earlier before going to a meeting in the next town. It was extremely unusual for me to be home at this time of day. Generally, I leave for my office around 6:20 am and return sometime in the early evening hours but on this particular day I had a meeting that began at 9:00 am at an office that was only about 15 minutes from home.

My wife, Dorene, also works full time. She generally goes to her office, which is only a mile and a half from our home, around 7:30am and returns around 4:00 pm. She either carries a lunch or buys something at the cafeteria. It is quite unusual for her to come home before the afternoon.

The fact that I did not have to leave as early as normal to begin my work day gave me a little more time to hang around my home and chit chat with my wife as she got ready for work. I vaguely remember her reply to my query about her day. She had mentioned something about going to the doctor's office for a check up because "that problem I've been having isn't going away as easily as it should."

Her problem was that she had been bothered by a urinary tract infection for a couple of weeks. Her primary care physician had given her one course of antibiotics to clear it up but the problem had recurred and after a short waiting period she was returning for her second course of treatment.

Truthfully, I didn't think too much about any of this and was hardly even paying attention. I had been aware of her urinary infection but thought it was on the mend. Besides, I am one of these husbands who doesn't want to know all the details when it comes to "women problems" and, particularly, when they have to do with anything below the belt line. These details I don't need to know and, frankly, my wife is the type of person who keeps such things to herself.

When I drove into my driveway and hit the button to open the garage door, I was surprised to see that my wife's car was in the garage. The thought had not even entered my mind that she was coming from a doctor's appointment. I know that she told me about the appointment but I had forgotten entirely.

As I entered our kitchen through the doorway from our cellar stairs that lead to the garage, Dorene's back was to me and she was standing by the kitchen table. I sort of matter-of-factly asked her, "What are you doing home?" She turned with a contorted face that I will never forget because it was filled with fear and sadness like I had never seen before and said, "I've got Cancer." Big tear drops were running down her cheeks.

I can't remember exactly the thoughts that I had at that particular instance but there were many all at once. But in spite of these thoughts, I instantly pulled her in my arms, kissed her wet cheek and held her tightly and remember saying to her, "Calm down, I love you and everything is going to be fine. We will get through this together and you will be just fine." Then I asked her to explain what had happened.

Apparently, she had not told me earlier in the day when she mentioned going back to the doctor's that it was a specialist that she was going to see. This doctor had been recommended by her primary care physician. Coincidentally, he had just moved his office from Boston, where he did a great deal of his work at Beth Israel Hospital to our home town. He said that most of his patients were from the suburbs and other than major surgeries, he could perform most of his procedures at a satellite, Beth, Israel, Deaconess Hospital that was located just down the street.

The primary care physician had referred Dorene to this urologist because, as I learned for the first time, she had discovered a little blood in her urine. I knew about the antibiotics and the fact that Doe(nickname) was having a recurrence, but she never told me about seeing the pink tinge in her urine that had prompted a repeat visit to primary care physician. And, she had, certainly not mentioned anything about the appointment with the urologist.

The urologist had performed a procedure called a cystoscopy. This involved taking a very thin wire with a microscopic camera lens on it and inserting it through the urethra up into the bladder. It allows the doctor to look and see what is going on. The procedure is relatively painless and doesn't take long. It can be done in the doctor's office with only a local anesthesia. The doctor, who Dorene seemed to like, had told her rather matter-of-factly that she had a cancerous tumor in her bladder and that it would have to be removed. They had made an appointment for the middle of the next week for us to go and see him so that we could discuss the next procedure.

Although I learned all of this later, at that particular point and time, all I was doing was calming Dorene down and learning the very basics: that she had cancer; that it was in her bladder; that she had undergone a procedure where they looked up into her bladder; that there was no doubt in the doctor's mind, and that we would be going in together to see him and learn more.

At this point, I need to divert a bit and tell you a bit more about myself. I am not a touchy-feely kind of guy. This is not to say that I am insensitive because I care greatly about how others think and feel and am troubled most when I believe that I have hurt someone's feelings. However, I was raised like a lot of other kids of Irish, working class, parents not to talk about the way things affect you inside and to just deal with them.

My wife is very similar in some ways, in that, she doesn't display a great deal of outward "neediness." She is not a high maintenance kind of person. However, having said that, she is entirely different from me emotionally. Her feelings are very real and are easily hurt. She is a kind, and empathetic person, and can bruise easily on the inside, although it may not be apparent to people from the outside. She is not one to talk to me about such bruises unless they are really bothering her, I sense them and offer my help.

Other than on these rare cases, we don't talk a lot about the things that are bothering us . . . . at least, not to each other. I do believe that Dorene has a network of friends with whom she would be able to discuss these types of things and probably does, but I don't pay a lot attention to it.

When I look back to the instant when my wife turned to me, I have vivid memories. I had never seen her as upset as she was. She tried not to cry but literally burst out with an outward display of both emotion and horror. I am actually made a bit uncomfortable even thinking about it now. And other than her declaration of the cancer, nothing was said immediately.

My reaction of instantly holding her in my arms and kissing her on the cheek was two things: it was an unusual gut reaction for me to have and it was absolutely the appropriate thing to do. Secondly, when I told her that I loved her and assured her that everything would be o.k. and that we would handle this together, it was the right thing to say and seemed to have an instant calming and soothing effect.

I remember getting this instant rush of emotion. I was scared, confused, angry, bewildered, and saddened all at once. It only lasted an instant but I was, for this instant, literally speechless. It may have really only lasted more like a second but I remember it clearly because I have never had this convergence of feelings in my life. It was almost like a white-out in my mind for that one second as my brain was bombarded with emotions that I normally don't have, or, at least, do a pretty good job of masking.

This went away as quickly as it came once I held my wife and assured her that things would be o.k. You see, this role of being the "provider" is one that I am far more comfortable doing. It is the way that I was raised.

However, I am still amazed by the fact that I did everything right at that particular moment of crisis. I am not bragging, by any means. In retrospect, I am pleased with myself, but still amazed. Maybe it was a natural reaction because I love my wife and have for our entire adult life. But believe me, it was a bit unusual for me to know what to say in an emotional crisis. Usually, I say the wrong thing and make things much worse.

This brings me to my first important revelation in the process of helping someone heal: you have to, and should, be demonstratively supportive to your loved one who is ill. I don't care whether you have been in the past or whether it makes you feel uncomfortable. It's no longer about you. It's all about doing everything that is within your power to help your loved one get better.

It's important for both your loved one and for you, to hear you say that you love them and care about them and for you to reassure him or her that everything will be o.k. My experience has shown me that this simple act of truth and open expression of love has helped both my wife and me. I think that sometimes I tell her that I love her just to hear her say, "I love you, too."

I will talk about this a bit later, but you, too, have been affected by your loved one's illness. All of the emotions that he or she has experienced, you have also to some degree. Providing any little tools that you can pick up here to help you deal with your particular crisis is my sole motivation for writing this book.

There is an incredible spiritual side to all of this as well. I've heard that many people have wondered how God can let bad things happen to good people. I don't know the answer to this and don't think it is really worth pondering. I only want to put my energies where they can do some good.

In the interest of transparency, I must admit, however, that I did have negative thoughts. In my wife's case, she is a very religious person with very strong beliefs. I don't know anybody who does more to help others. She is as kind a person as I have ever met. She gives charitably continually and is always ready to support any person in need whether it be spiritually, emotionally, or financially. She goes to church regularly and prayer is a big part of her life. But, she still got cancer.

I don't know the "whys" of all this. I do think that there is a God and I don't think that He had anything to do with my wife getting cancer. I just think that cancer and other diseases are thing that have evolved in mankind and that my wife is no different than hundreds of thousands, in fact, millions of others, who have suffered from them in some way, shape or form. If He had anything to do with it, my religion teaches me that it would probably be for some good that we have yet to comprehend.

The only thing special about my wife or your loved one getting cancer is that we love them and care about them! That makes it take on a whole new enormity to us. It represents a threat to the very thing we cherish most in life and throws a wrench into the works of our human psychological makeup. But, regardless of your religion or whoever or whatever you believe to be your source of spiritual power (I choose God), He, She, or It has nothing to do with your loved one getting cancer. It is a malady that is affecting mankind.

However, I do believe whole heartedly that there is a source of spiritual power that helps both the sick person and those that surround him or her. Again, because I am not a theologian and not steeped in knowledge in this regard, I am not sure how it all works. I will leave that to others. But, if you learn to listen to that inner voice, or that gut-feeling that we all get from time to time, I think that you, too, will come to appreciate this. I believe that the source is from God. You can believe it comes from someone or something else, but I am certain that it is there and that both you and your sick loved one will benefit from it.

I don't think for one moment that it was a "coincidence" that I hung around my house a bit that morning and chit-chatted with my wife. Similarly, that my meeting was close enough to my home that I would swing by to pick up the papers that I had, "coincidentally," forgotten that morning or even that I "instinctively" knew how to act or what to say at that moment of crisis. The fact that the doctor had just moved his office to our town so that it was only moments away from our home and that we both arrived home that morning at the same time are other unusual "coincidences." If you aren't a believer, fine with me, as I am not a crusader, but I have thought about much of my experience with both amazement and wonderment. I have come to appreciate that these coincidences are from this source of power. If you allow yourself to see them, to contemplate them, and to feel them, you will discover that they are happening to you, too. I suggest that you give it a try.

All that you have to do is remain open to recognizing some good things that are happening along the way. It is so easy to be stricken by the scary and bad things that you can easily overlook some things that are simple that didn't necessarily have to happen the way that they did. What if I hadn't forgotten my papers that morning? What if my meeting had been in the next town? I am grateful that I was able to be with my wife shortly after her getting this very scary news and don't think that it happened by accident.

My wife has often told me over the years that fear is the absence of faith and that faith is the absence of fear. This makes great sense to me. To further the equation, I believe that to the extent that you have a lot of one, you will have less of the other. I believe that we can "tune in" to certain signs and receive help in replacing fear with faith.

Lastly, as you go through the journey of helping your loved one deal with their health situation, try to stay in the present. Deal with what is at any particular point in time. Yes, you will research and learn all about the disease. But the only thing that really matters is the current situation and getting through it.

If your mind is like mine and millions of others, it allows you to wander off in fear as you learn about complications and various stages of the disease. This is natural enough but it does very little in terms of keeping you positive and dealing with the present. Try to remember this throughout out your entire journey. Stay in the present!

Like so many things in life, this is more easily said than done. However, by thinking about it now, you may be able to ward off going to places that you need not be in the future. Remember to deal with "what is", not with "what could be!"

Chapter Two

Knowledge is Power

Needless to say, I didn't go to work that afternoon. I stayed home, comforted Dorene and began my research.

I understand that all people are different. I tend to be a person who deals with a crisis like this, particularly one with which I am totally unfamiliar, by trying to learn as much as I possibly can. My wife is not like this. In her case, perhaps because she knows the way I am, she doesn't want to know all the ugly facts, particularly when they could involve her. She leaves that to me and trusts that I will familiarize myself with them.

This was startling news to us. We all wanted to know the prognosis. We wanted to know if this would kill her. Neither of us brought up this nasty subject but, you can be sure, it was on our minds.

That first day, I read and read and read. Much of the information that I read, I knew that I would have to reread in order to fully comprehend. However, before I went to bed that night, I had gained enough knowledge to tell my wife that I, honestly, believed that this cancer would not kill her.

My advice to you is to get as much information as you possibly can about your loved one's illness. The internet is incredible. I read and I read and I read. I looked up all of the terms, even looked up their pronunciation and Latin roots so that I could be more conversant with medical folks and less apt to forget them.

There is just so much to learn that a lay person really only discovers how much they don't know. But, I do believe that the knowledge you gain will be helpful to your loved one and will provide him or her with a better chance of survival. You need to acquire, at least, basic knowledge in order to help in the future.

I wanted to be able to understand what to expect. My research enabled me. I read the mortality rates and the treatment procedures. I learned about the most likely surgeries and the options that would be presented. Then I learned about these various options and the risks associated with each.

I knew that Dorene would ultimately have to make the decisions and that my job would be to help her. In the end, all of these decisions had to be made by her but I was able to give her a lot of the information she needed. Sometimes it was just a case of "translating" what the medical people were saying into terms that make sense to the rest of us.

Another suggestion that I would give to anybody going through this is to write down every single question that you come across. If you find the answers yourself while researching than just cross them off the list. But keep a list of questions. Write them down on paper. When the time comes to speak to the doctors, don't let them go until your questions have been fully answered. You will find that even when doing this, you will still come up with other questions among yourselves after the consultations. In this sense, your list of questions is a living document that is continually changing and evolving as questions get crossed out and new ones added.

Again, all folks are different. I am not troubled by information. As a matter of fact, I prefer to get it all: the good news and the bad. My wife is different to me in this regard, as well. She does not want to know much of the information. If she doesn't need to know it, she would rather not.

She also gets "creeped-out" by things easier than me. I learned to respect this early on and to give her only the information that she wanted to know or that I felt was essential to a decision that she would have to make in the future.

After all, she is brighter than me and she knows how to use the internet as well. I suspected that she did a bit of this early on until it bothered her too much to continue. It's one thing to read this type of stuff when you are unfamiliar with it. But it is an entirely different animal when you are reading about things that might happen to you and your body.

Slowly, and only as my wife wished, we would talk about different issues. I always presented the information truthfully but with as positive approach as I could. I was the guy that likes to talk about this stuff and I had to keep reminding myself that this wasn't about me, it was about my wife, her feelings and her body. I guarantee that you, too, will have to remain ever vigilant to this. You must put your loved one's needs and desires above your own as it is no longer about you. It's the other person that is sick and needs help. You will end up doing just fine.

One of the first things that comes up is who are we going to tell and who is going to be the one doing the telling. My wife made it clear that she didn't want anyone other than my children to know until she knew what was going on and that wouldn't be until the middle of the next week at the very earliest. As it turned out, we had to wait a couple more weeks before we really knew.

Dorene ended up deciding that we should tell our sons. I have two grown sons. One of them lives nearby and we see him all the time. The other lives in Las Vegas. But, the two boys talk daily. They are not kids any more, one is nearly 40 and the other is 36. But, nevertheless, this kind of news is shocking to anybody, never mind when we are talking about a woman who was a health nut working out every day and watching everything that she ate.

My wife didn't want anyone else to know until she had all the information. Believe it or not, this is a tough thing that you will have to respect. Looking back, I felt bad for myself and I wanted my friends to know. I suspect that I wanted to tell them not because of their relationship with my wife, but, I think, because I wanted someone to feel bad for me because I was really hurting inside and masking it pretty well. I don't think that I knew this at the time but it is pretty clear to me now. The caregiver is hurting as well. But, the big difference is that you as a care giver will get over it. So, if you're feeling that way, just get over it!

In the end, I respected my wife's wishes and you should too! You can go and get a pat on the back any time that you want it once the news breaks but at the beginning you really need to respect the feelings of the person who is sick and get over yourself! I did this and am proud that I did.

Telling my boys was easy for me to do as we are very close. Dorene sobbed when I told the first son. He was present because he lives nearby. My wife cried when I told him. He's like me and asked a lot of questions that we were able to answer in a positive way. Dorene asked me to tell him for no other reason than she was unable to tell anyone without crying. The more she loved them, the more she would cry.

Again, my tendency is to want to blurt out the details and to solicit discussion and conversation. In retrospect, a part of this might have again been selfish desire to have someone with whom I could talk over all this scary information. My wife is not at all like this. She didn't want to hear the details herself and didn't want anyone else to know any more than they had to know. In the case of my sons, she wanted us to be candid, not to scare them and to answer as many questions as we could.

My second son was easier to tell because his brother had already called him and spilled the beans. He, too, had a lot of questions. Both of my kids are very bright. I don't doubt for one second that they were on the websites themselves in no time.

My Las Vegas son called me the next day with a referral. One of his employee's father, as it turned out, was a respected Doctor at MD Anderson Cancer Center in Houston. The son had already spoken to his Dad and given me his cell phone number so that I could call him with questions. I held off but said that I would when the time came and I needed some professional outside advice.

I also immediately went to work on checking out our urologist. I read his bio. I also checked him out with a state agency to find out if there had ever been any complaints filed against him. Dorene and I used all of our resources to make sure that he was the right man for the job. As it turned out, he was also an adjunct professor at Harvard Medical School where he taught the very procedure that Dorene ended up having. Dorene had a nurse friend check him out at the hospital and was told that he was the guy that they would recommend if asked by friends for a good urologist/oncologist.

I used every resource available to us. A neighbor is a doctor and his wife is a nurse. I was able to explain to them our situation and they were able to give us some really helpful advice about research and to recommend certain courses of action to help us gain information. All of this was processed and proved helpful in making our final decisions.

You should do this as well. If you know anybody even related to medical field, get their advice and opinions. This is probably all new information to you. Any help that you can find is worth getting. Sometimes good advice can come from the least expected sources.

So armed with my legal pad of questions, we went to meet with the Doctor for our first consultation. He was a nice man but didn't pull any punches when it came to telling us about his suspicions and in letting us know what he believed had to be done next.

We both listened attentively as he explained all of this. I then began with my questions from my list. But, the truth be told, he had answered most of them with his very thorough explanation. I immediately agreed with my wife's positive assessments of him.

The next procedure would have to be a day surgery at the suburban hospital. It was called a trasurethal resection and basically it meant the tumor would be accessed the same way as it was with the "scope" but that they would scrape out a bit or all of it and send it to the lab for tests and classification. I had read about all this and knew that it was standard procedure. This surgery was scheduled for a week and a half later at the local hospital.

Nine days later she went to the local satellite hospital of the bigger Boston brand for her surgery. The urologist had originally told us that it would probably be a day surgery and that Dorene would go home that night. However, she was admitted overnight as she was very ill. It seems that anesthesia and drugs, in general, don't settle well with her. She was very ill.

The drug of choice did little to abate the nausea that she was experiencing but there was an older drug that finally got the situation under control. I wrote the name of this drug down. This proved to be of great value later when she went in for the major surgery.

At this same time, one of the nurses told us about a patch that could be put on the day before surgery that would help alleviate some of the nausea created by the anesthesia. I wrote this down on my list to discuss with the doctor prior to any further surgery that might be needed.

Oddly enough, two days prior to this first procedure, Dorene was going out with a lifelong girlfriend and with her older sister for a "girls night out." Even though she had the weight of the situation on her mind, she didn't tell them. Her older sister is very helpful and caring but tends to get very involved when these types of things happen. In Dorene's family, telling her would be like sending a telegram to everybody in the extended family and every friend of Dorene's. She didn't want to have to worry about others at this time and wasn't ready to chance that happening, so she didn't say a word.

During these two days, my wife's phone was ringing off the hook. The older sister knew something was up. She is incredibly perceptive when it comes to the family and she had been unable to reach her sister and had tried both house and cell phone.

She knew that it was very strange that I had gone to the movies with Dorene and her younger brother the night before our surgery (something that I would almost never do). She put two and two together and would not stop calling because she couldn't find her sister.

Finally, because Dorene was ill, in the hospital and didn't want to be bothered anymore(by now, the elder sister had all six siblings and the parents involved), she finally spilled the beans to her sister and asked her to give her cover and not to tell anyone. The sister respected her wishes but demanded to be kept informed.

The urologist called us in a few days later and gave us the bad news. The cancer was very invasive and had to come out. He suggested a radical cystectomy.

Again, we pulled out all the stoppers when it came to the research. All the while, I wrote down my questions. I spoke to the Doctor from MD Anderson and another doctor who practiced in this area who was referred by a surgeon friend of ours.

We had a consult with our urologist who told us his reasons for the cystectomy and discussed the various options available to her. He thought that someone in Doene's shape would be home in 7-10 days and back to work in a couple of months.

We asked lots of questions about the various options regarding this procedure and kept finding ourselves, both of us did, coming back to the same conclusion. The on-going research and the list of questions were all answered at this consultation. We left the meeting without any grave questions. Our research had given us the confidence to know what we believed had to be done and the doctor concurred. So, we scheduled the surgery.

We still had the matter of telling Dorene's elderly parents who were vacationing at her brother's house across the country. As good fortune would have it, the older sister was out there, too. She is married to a nice guy who happens to be a nurse and who has a great way with her parents. For that matter, his knowledge and familiarity with all things medical proved very calming and informative to all of us throughout the ordeal.

So what we did was call one day when he was there, knowing that he would have a calming and grounding effect. The older sister had already told the parents that Dorene would be calling with some news (this added to the drama that is so typical in our family). We called and assured them that everything would be ok.

I think that our planning with the brother in law worked, as he reassured them that it was serious but that Dorene seemed to have a good handle on it. So, that planning went well and the parents, although gravely concerned, handled it well. Of course, from then on all cell phones were ringing and the cat was out of the bag. The whole world knew!

At the end of the day, a bit of planning on what and how to tell loved ones is probably a good idea. It takes some of the drama and worry out of it as everybody has the right to be concerned because they love the sick person.

We believed that being honest, without a lot of the gorier details, was the right way to go in telling friends and family about the cisis. It makes little sense to sugar coat too much because then they won't believe you. Simple truth, here as in most things in life, worked for us.

But the lesson that we learned here is that you must, yet again, respect the wishes of the sick person. As tough as I think that I am, I wanted others to know so that they would feel some sympathy for me because I was feeling pretty bad for myself. I learned to recognize this self-pity and fought it off every time it would come creeping into my psyche because I know that it would do no good at all. All it does is fill you with negativity and make an ugly situation seem even uglier.

As expected, my wife's parents cancelled their vacation and came home so that they could be supportive of their daughter during the surgery. Her brother from California also came home so that he could be present during the surgery. They respected and understood our concerns that there would be no sense in them visiting for a few days until Dorene was able to see them. My job was to keep them informed as they were just as anxious as I was. After all, this was their daughter and sister.

Chapter Three

Surgery

In mid March, we showed up at the hospital at the designated time. Dorene was admitted after all of the paper work was completed. She was sent to a pre-surgery room in the Beth, Israel, Deaconess Hospital in Boston. The nurses in this area, in spite of their rather hectic environment, were very supportive.

For someone who has never been in this situation, it can be a bit over whelming. There is very little privacy and there are many other patients who are all awaiting their turn in the Operating Room, or OR as it is called.

There are many consults with various medical personnel. Medical histories are painstakingly reviewed, over and over again. Originally, I was asked to wait in the waiting room. Once the pre-surgery room became relatively quiet as the different patients were wheeled into surgery, I was allowed to visit with my wife as she awaited her turn.

The professionalism of the staff was very apparent. They were comforting and reassuring. The Anesthesiologist came and did her last interview. She had arranged for Dorene to wear the patch the night before that had been suggested by the nurse at the satellite hospital.

This entire procedure is one of checking and rechecking various check lists and asking all the appropriate questions.

At this point, I was aware because of our research of the importance of antibiotics being administered in a timely fashion just prior to surgery. Again, I would urge any loved one to become familiar with all of these details as your job of advocate, perhaps the most important role that you will play, has already begun.

I was able to inquire about the antibiotics and was assured that the intravenous drip had the antibiotics in it. As small as this may seem, it is of critical importance and I was confident that Dorene was being treated in a fashion that was following all of the protocols with which we had become familiar.

The last visit was from her surgeon. He was very confident and reassuring.

Never before had I experienced the wisdom of my wife's teaching as in this situation. You are completely at the mercy of professionals that you really don't know all that well. Yes, your research may tell you that they are competent and all things should go well. But, in the back of your mind you are aware that there can be problems. Fear is, indeed, the opposite of faith. And, whether faith comes from beliefs rooted in religion or from knowledge, or from a combination of both, it is put to the test in these situations.

We were prepared both emotionally and spiritually and were as comfortable as could be expected.

The staff came to wheel Dorene into the OR. I gave her a kiss on the forehead and told her that I loved her and reassured her that she would be fine. They wheeled her into the operating room and I went to the waiting area.

Joining me in the waiting room was my son and my brother in law from California. In retrospect, I was pleased to have other people with me. Of course the wait is long and seems even longer than the hours would let you believe. We were able to converse, sometimes about Dorene and her situation, sometimes about other things totally unrelated. The six hours in the waiting room seems like a blur to me now. I know that the company I had with me helped and would recommend to anyone that they bring friends or family with them as this can be tough time and is better spent with others.

Eventually, her surgeon came out and told us that everything went well. Dorene's physical shape had aided him and he told us that he was very pleased with how things went. He explained that I would be allowed in the recovery room in about an hour and that after a period of time there, Dorene would be brought up to her room.

In about an hour, I called the recovery room and was told that they would let me know when I could come up. My son and brother in law went home, knowing that things went well. I used this time to call her parents and her sister so that they could call other family members. In about two hours, I received the call and proceeded to the recovery room.

Dorene was barley awake and heavily sedated. She looked good albeit very tired. She had IV's in her arms. An NG tube in her nose that was connected to a vacuum pump and a bag connected by a tube to her that was filling with bloody bodily fluids.

I gave her a kiss, told her that I loved her, and reassured her that all of the medical personnel had told me that things went remarkably well.

I think that I did a pretty good job of not being startled by all of this medical "stuff". I tried my hardest, as I did in many other situations during this ordeal, to put my discomfort aside and to act comfortable around these sorts of things with which I was almost totally unfamiliar. I believe that my comfort level made Dorene feel a bit more comfortable. She continued to rest as some of the sedation slowly wore off.

The nurses in this area were also extremely supportive and kind. As the sedation wore off, Dorene had moments of sadness. I was told that sedation can have the effect of increasing the emotions. She was already emotional as her body had been violated in a way that would alter it forever. However, both she and I knew that this was a necessary step in ridding her of the cancer that just hours before was threatening her life.

At different times, the tears came uncontrollably and rolled down her cheeks. The nurses were very loving and told her that it was ok to cry as she had been through so much. At the same time, they also assured her that she would be fine, to remain strong, and to keep in the present.

As I mentioned before, staying in the present is another bit of wisdom that is an essential take away from our experience. I believe that all of us caregivers have a tendency to project our concerns for our loved one onto our thoughts of how they must be feeling. Although this is natural, I suggest that it is counterproductive when dwelled upon.

The truth is that you do not necessarily know what your loved one is thinking or feeling at any time. It is not about you, but about them. They are entitled to their thoughts and concerns and your job is to be steady in your resolve to help them get better. In other words, you have to suck it up, cast your fears aside, and put on a straight and loving face that will help prevent natural fears from taking grasp of you, and eventually, your loved one. This is far easier said than done but with diligence, I suspect that you will be able to do it and will even surprise yourself with your resolve: fear is the opposite of faith!

Even if you are filled with fear, fake it until you make it and this, too, shall pass!

Eventually, Dorene was wheeled up to her room. The room was a semi-private room with nobody else in it. I had requested, in advance, a private room and was disappointed when I was told that none were available. Apparently, the floor was very busy as another floor was being remodeled. They did have one private room available but had to keep it open in case a person with an infectious disease needed it.

I think that a couple of points here deserve mentioning. First of all, if you can afford the additional charges for a private room, try to get one. Secondly, your advocacy for you loved one is continual from the day of diagnosis. I was determined to get a private room and made sure that every, single, nurse knew it. I did it in a very nice way so that they, too, could become advocates for us.

Nurses are very special people. They are the ones that give the care in hospitals. Doctors make the decisions but nurses give the care. They can be extremely harried at different times. I made sure to let every one of them know just how much I appreciated them caring for my wife. I found out about their families and their personal lives. I was very kind to them even when I had to be assertive as I knew that they were the messengers between us and the powers that be.

Finally, on this first night, my wife was resting peacefully and I went home. I had spent 15 hours in the hospital and had witnessed my brave wife go through a great deal. I went home and slept in my in own bed.

Although I will not give a day by day of my wife's stay in the Beth, Israael, Deaconess Hospital of Boston, I will tell you that on day two she was quite ill. She had a terrible problem with nausea. They tried everything and she never really got over it throughout her entire stay. Nothing ever really seemed to work. Fortunately, we had written down the name of the drug that worked during the smaller procedure and they used it with some success.

I think that the narcotics made her ill. She was vomiting on day two when she had another person admitted to her room. In the afternoon, the roommate had company that could have cared less about my wife's condition. They brought in fried chicken that smelled the whole room up and acted like they were at an outside park rather than in a hospital room that was shared by someone else who was very ill. I continued to let the nurses know of my unhappiness and asked them to check on a private room.

My wife never really got much better from here. The doctor came by and they did some x-rays. Apparently the x-rays showed a problem.

During the major surgery that Dorene had undergone, her bladder was removed and a new bladder was created out of a part of intestine. The tubes that run from the kidneys to the bladder, uretas, are reconnected to the new bladder and stents are put in them to aid healing and to prevent leaking at the connection points.

For some reason, these stents had to be removed. They had slipped and if not removed, we were told, they could cause some serious blockages. This is a very simple procedure and is painless.

On the third day, a seasoned nurse came in and removed the stents. You could tell that she had been around for a while. She seemed surprised when these stents were removed because she said they were too short. Again, the purpose of the stents is to create a continuum between the kidneys and the new bladder that had been constructed where my wife's bladder had been removed. This prevents leakage from various places where the uretas are reconnected to this new bladder.

For some reason or another, these stents, which are suppose to remain for about a week, were being removed approximately 48 hours later.

We also befriended a nurse who was working 3-11 on the third day. My wife's condition had continued to worsen. The nausea had not relented and the lady in the other half of the room was doing projectile vomiting and making sounds that would make anyone sick. My wife was really suffering and not recovering the way that everyone had hoped. She was miserable.

By now, my wife's condition had worsened to the point that I was sleeping in her room. I would continue to do so until her release some 23 days later. The day nurse stuck her head in the door around 12:30 am and said that she had stuck around to do some paperwork but that a private room was available and that I could have it if we wanted to move now. Even though my wife was very sick and had finally fallen asleep, I decided that privacy would be better and we moved to a room that we would stay in for another 24 days.

Had I not been around, and had I not befriended this particular nurse, I believe that we would never have gotten a private room. This is an example of why the patient needs an advocate present all of the time. Don't think that it will be different at your hospital. This is one of the best hospitals in the country. If you don't look out for your loved one, chances are that nobody else will.

You see, without an advocate for the patient, everybody is busy doing their jobs. The nurses like it to be quiet because they are so harried when it is not. If I weren't in that room on that particular night and had I not talked to the nurses about the private room earlier in the evening, they never would have taken it upon themselves to move us. They would have enjoyed the quiet of the evening and not done anything extra. My wife would have had to continue to put up with the sounds and smells of another sick person.

My stars were aligned in a particular way and, yes, this was another coincidence: our friendly day nurse had stayed late to do paper work and had heard the nurses over talking about a new admission going into the private room. She decided to act in spite of the fact that she was an hour and a half late getting off her shift and home to her family.

Providing around the clock presence is very difficult for most families. However, you should try to be present or to have someone present as much as possible Your patient, at least when they are very sick, needs constant care. The only way that you can assure it is by being present, paying attention, and speaking up.

For example, the IV machines are always buzzing. This sets off an alarm at the nurse station, a light outside the room and your nurse is sent to your room. Most always these are of a non-emergency nature. They are either because a particular IV has run out or there is a crimp or air bubble in the line.

These alarms can be very annoying to a person who is riddled with nausea and headaches or if the patient has finally nodded off to sleep. Generally speaking, the nurses are annoyed by these things and are in no hurry to quiet them because they have more pressing things to do.

I observed the nurses and learned what the different alarms meant and how they quieted them down. If the alarm went off and the nurse didn't respond, I would go out to the nurses' station to let them know. If they still didn't respond, I would take the initiative to shut it off and then I would stand outside the room and look for our nurse so that I could run her down and get her to deal with the issue.

Again, this may seem like a very simple thing and you may think that I sound like I am a complainer. I am not. I just wanted the best possible treatment for my suffering wife.

I also used the grease board in my wife's room to record every medicine that she took and other vital issues of concern. I did this throughout her stay. I knew the limitations on the medicine and was able to suggest others based upon the graphs that I kept. This sounds foolish, but I didn't want to have to rely on the nurse coming on duty to have to read the log and be aware of things that had happened during a prior shift. You need to pay attention to this.

Sometimes, something that you think is rather significant could have happened during a shift. The nurse on duty may have not witnessed it or may not have been impressed and might not have written it up in the log. The information that you can provide to the incoming nurses may be critical to your loved one. For example, perhaps you have noticed that a particular narcotic was more effective or less effective. Or maybe you noticed a more adverse reaction to one drug than another. Or that there was a timeline issue of which nobody else seemed aware.

Writing down and recording everything is so important. In many cases, the medical folks will be aware of your observations. But, don't sell yourself short, in many cases you may provide critical observations that nobody else has seen that may be significant to your loved one's healing.

So far I have talked primarily about communications with the nursing staff. Overall, I would say that nurses represent the best side of the medical system. They show the most compassion and are the people who give direct care to the patient. They are responsive and, I think, appreciative of your efforts because they help with the overall care of the patient.

This is not to say that the doctors care any less. I am sure that the doctors care as much. I know that our surgeon, certainly, did. However, there is a hierarchy in the hospital system that is counterproductive to good care. The doctors are the bosses and the nurses are the workers.

The nurses take their marching orders from the doctors. They report back to the doctors and the doctors make all the decisions. Communications are incredibly poor between the different levels of this hierarchy and the patients.

The surgeon is the big boss and he leads the team. Beth, Israel, Deaconess Hospital is a teaching hospital and the team consists of various doctors who are all residents with different years of experience. Whatever the surgeon says goes and there is very little disagreement shown to the patients. The lead resident is in charge of the other residents and, again, they are very careful in making sure that no dissenting opinions are allowed to be witnessed by the patients. Only by asking a lot of direct questions to the doctors when they are around, and to the nurses when they are not, can you get to the truth of what they are actually thinking, particularly when there are problems.

Keeping your list of questions and observations is critical to your loved one's care. Do not be afraid or uncomfortable about asking all of your questions whenever you get the chance. Don't let them leave without your thoughts being expressed. Only then can you even begin to get the information that you need.

Our experience showed us that unless you ask questions, you will know next to nothing about your loved one's condition. The doctors, or the team as they were known at Beth Israel, will give you no information. If you find yourself having questions after you have been graced by their presence, you probably haven't asked enough questions.

In my opinion, the doctors do not want to be bothered by you, the advocate. They want to be, instead, absolutely in charge and to always project an air of confidence even when any observer can see that things are going drastically wrong. This is exactly what happened in the case of my wife. Mistakes were made, there was some finger pointing, and I will never know who did what wrong . . . . but there were many things done wrong.

Chapter Four

The Hospital Stay: One Crisis after another

My wife's condition continued to worsen in her first week in the hospital. They were totally unable to get a handle on her problems and she was getting worse, hour by hour, in front of my very eyes.

First there was the issue of the NG tube. The NG tube is common after abdominal surgery. It goes through the nose, down the esophagus and into the stomach. It vacuums out stomach bile that would otherwise make the patient ill. It is very a very uncomfortable apparatus and causes pain.

In my wife's case this pain was extreme and continued to get worse. She was sick. Her stomach was distended and getting bigger and harder by the hours. She had a fever every day. They sent her for CT Scans to see what was wrong.

One day the pain from the NG tube became excruciating. There had been no bile coming out of the drainage tube into the vacuum container. She told the nurse that she was getting pains shooting up through her ears and the side of her head. The reply was that nobody likes the NG tube and it does make people uncomfortable.

Again, this is where an advocate is needed. I know my wife. I know that a little discomfort would not make her ask me to get the nurse. I know that her pain was real and excruciating. She does not exaggerate such things.

I asked to have the doctor come in and see us. They reported back that they had spoken to the doctor and that he said pain medication should work. I politely said that this was unacceptable, that the medication was not helping, and that I wanted to see the doctor.

A resident showed up and they decided to take the NG tube out as it hadn't produced any bile in hours. They did this and my wife immediately had relief, not from the nausea but from the pains in her head.

I learned from the nurses that the urine output from her new bladder was pretty good on one side but that on the other it was very poor. Her right side was doing pretty well but the left side was not. This was the same side that the seasoned nurse had notice the short stent.

Her belly continued to grow and the drainage bulb that was connected by a tube into her incision area, the Jackson Pratt or JP as it is called, was not collecting many fluids. This is like a basting bulb that creates a bit of suction and takes fluids from the body cavity at the point of the incision via the tube that goes directly into the body cavity.

She continued to suffer and was very sick. Then, as good fortune will have it, that same, older, seasoned nurse, the one that had taken out the stents a week earlier, came by to change the apparatus that was part of her new urinary system. She looked at my wife's belly and exclaimed that her belly was distended and that she must have a "leak." Then, she went out and talked to the doctors at the nurses' station.

Shortly thereafter, probably within a couple of hours, the nurse on duty noticed that the JP drain in her belly was full with urine and emptied it. It immediately filled up again. She emptied it only to have it fill up a third time, immediately.

She went out to the nurses' station and then came back and replaced the bulb that was connected to the drainage tube to a foley (plastic bag). Immediately, nearly three liters of urine came out of my wife's body cavity. Keep in mind, this wasn't from her bladder or kidneys this was from the inside of her body cavity where there was not suppose to be any urine to speak of other than that tiny bit that would leak from the connection of the ureta to the new bladder. No wonder she was so sick. The older, experienced, nurse was correct: there was a leak!

Shortly after this, our surgeon dropped by and said that the CT Scan had shown a leak. He had been on vacation so we had not seen him much up to this point. He said that on occasion the stents slip down and have to be removed and that he believed that removing them had caused a leak on the left side.

He suggested a procedure that would divert the urine from her body by placing two nephrostomy tubes into the kidneys through my wife's back. This would allow two bags to capture the urine directly from the kidneys thereby facilitating the healing of the uretas at the new connections at the new bladder and stopping the leaks. The procedure was scheduled with radiology.

My wife was very, very sick. She was nauseous and in great pain. I went with her as she was wheeled to the radiology department to do this procedure. I made the transportation people go very slowly. This is important.

On other trips they had gone too fast, hitting bumps and wheeling around corners and this had made my wife sick to her stomach. The motion, combined with the intense nausea, fever, and sickness had caused her to get sick. As simple as this sounds, I made them go slow. I did it in a nice way and was very complimentary to their "driving" and understanding. I got to know the transport people by their first names and would greet them in the hallways. They slowed down and it made a huge difference to a very sick woman. If I were not there, they would have just dealt with the resulting vomit. Again, you must always be the vigilant advocate. Don't assume anything and don't be afraid to make demands. Your observations are very important to your loved one's experience.

The process of getting those tubes into the kidneys is done by radiologists as they have to use x-rays during the process as they thread a long needle past nerves and arteries in order to make a direct hit into the kidneys. The patient has to lie on his or her stomach as they go in through the back. My wife was sick and was not sure that she would be able to stand being on her stomach. It was still very distended. They went ahead with the procedure and I waited outside as I was told it would take about an hour.

After about two hours and fifteen minutes, the kind operating nurse stuck her head out to give me an update. She said that she didn't know if they would be able to finish as my wife was about at "the end of her rope." She said that they had one tube in and that my wife had been vomiting the whole time and that she was frazzled. I asked her how much more time would be required and she told me about 15 minutes. I told her to continue as I didn't want my wife to have to face this horrible experience again as it is done with just a relaxing drug and local anesthetic.

They completed the procedure and allowed me to go in and see Dorene in the OR as they were cleaning up. Dorene just rolled her eyes, completely exhausted and said something to the effect that she did not want to do that again. I noticed that the bags that were hooked up to the new nephrostomy tubes coming out of her back were already collecting urine.

The whole idea of this procedure was to create a urinary diversion, taking the urine out of the body and allowing the body to heal. It worked and the urine was filling these two bags. This was after about a week in the hospital and I will tell you that I immediately noticed Dorene looking better, in spite of the horrendous procedure that she had just undergone. The urine was no longer going into her body cavity and making her sick. She now had two Foleys (plastic drainage bags) connected to the two nephrostomy tubes, another connected by a tube to her new bladder, and a JP tube coming from her stomach.

All of this time, I should say, Dorene had not eaten any food. She was being fed by an IV as her intestine had been operated on during the major surgery when a piece of it was used to create a new bladder. Although she was showing signs of improvement, she was still incredibly nauseous every, single, minute of the day and night. They were never able to control her nausea. She felt better but was in pain from the tubes going into her back and into her kidneys.

The game plan was to give the connections a couple of days to heal and then to block off the nephrostomy drainage tubes one at time without removing them. This would force the urine back out through the kidneys, down through the uretas and out the new bladder. By measuring the input of fluids and the output through the bladder, the medical people would be able to determine whether or not the leak had been repaired.

After a few days of continued suffering incredible nausea every minute of the day, they did this only to find that the right side seemed to be ok but the left side was not producing enough urine through the bladder. They suspected that they still had a leak which was later confirmed by a CT Scan. They would have to try something else.

I asked the surgeon the next game plan and he told me that they would use the nephrostomy tubes as an entrance into the kidneys and that they would "snake" a wire through them, down the uretas and into the new bladder. Next, they intended to pull a stent or sleeve over the wire from the kidneys all the way into the new bladder or conduit as it was called. This would create an uninterrupted channel from the kidneys to the bladder and would ensure that there would be no leak. Additionally, these stents would, at the same time, promote healing at the connections of the uretas to the bladder. The stents could be removed very easily after everything was found to be working well.

All of this made great sense to me. I had read all about the urinary tract and this seemed completely logical. My only doubts were their ability to do this successfully and whether or not the connection would ever stop leaking.

Of course, I also had doubts about what had caused the original stents not to work. The older nurse said that they were too short. The surgeon said that they had slipped down. Another medical professional that was involved told us it was the surgeon's fault. I didn't care who was at "fault" all I wanted was for my wife to get better and I was pleased with this course of action.

To the doctor's credit, they explained to me that medical people focus on the problems at hand. Energy spent on determining what went wrong does little to help the patient. They treat symptoms. I agreed with their wisdom.

Our confidence in the hospital was waning with good reason. Dorene wasn't getting better. Someone had done something wrong.

Another time, she had been wheeled down to radiology for a procedure. The doctors were convinced that she had a pocket of urine in her that was draining. They thought that this was making her nauseous. They said that they could see the urine in the CT Scans.

This procedure would involve sticking a long needle through her buttocks into this pocket of urine in her body cavity and then extracting it with the syringe. She would be very sore afterwards because of all the muscle that they would have to go through.

After about an hour, they came out and said that they had not done it. They had three radiologists who all concurred that there was not pocket of urine. The pocket that the doctors had determined needed to be drained was urine in her new bladder that was not in the exact same place as her old bladder! Do you wonder that our confidence waned?

Radiology would have to do this new procedure also. We were told that Dorene would not be in much pain during the procedure. She was given something to calm her down and was wheeled, again very slowly, down to the radiology department where she was to have the procedure.

This time, the procedure was completed on time. Dorene came out unscathed and we went back up to her room. Shortly thereafter, the radiologist who had briefed us on the procedure showed up and said how beautifully everything went. He, himself, had done the left side. It took a bit of time but went in beautifully. His partner had done the right side and had it in very quickly. He explained that you can see it on the CT Scan as you are doing it and that everything went perfectly. This is the same doctor who had found the leak on the first CT Scan.

Both Dorene and I were relieved and felt that we were on the road to recovery. At this point, she had been in the hospital for nearly two weeks and had been through absolute hell. We knew that some mistake had been made or at least that something hadn't gone as it should. At the same time, we were hopeful that things would get better. Getting that urine out of her body cavity had shown us a little light at the end of the tunnel. Now, we were just hoping that they could just get these tube hooked up again so that the new bladder would work.

However she didn't get better. She felt sicker than ever. When they attempted to block off the nephrostomy tubes with the intention of forcing the urine out of the bladder, something seemed to be wrong and she got instantly sicker.

She knew something was wrong and asked that the nephrostomy tubes be opened immediately. She had an unusual sensation, was getting sicker by the minute and just knew that something was wrong!

I was very worried because I, too, knew something was wrong. This was like the gang that couldn't shoot straight but my wife's health and even life was at stake!

I remember having a conversation with one of the medical professionals that I had befriended. I suggested a meeting, like we might have in the business world, with all the doctors and me. I said that I would sign a statement that I wouldn't sue anyone but that I wanted to know their honest opinions about the problems that we continued to experience. I knew that things weren't working, that different people were pointing fingers at others, and that my wife was getting sicker by the minute.

I was reminded about the hierarchy that exists at the hospital when I suggested this to our new friend. I was told that this might work in a business setting but that it would never work at the hospital. When I asked why I was told that the surgeon would be the first to speak and then everybody would just nod their heads in agreement. Like it or not, that is the way that it is. There is an unofficial "code of silence" that exists within the hospital setting.

As chance will happen, another coincidence happened. My professional life puts me in touch with politicians on a regular basis.

One of the local politicians had heard about my wife's condition and called to ask if his office could be of any assistance.

My wife doesn't particularly care for the political process. Furthermore, she dislikes me involving politicians for anything. For this reason I declined the offer but thanked them for their concern. I wasn't even sure if this person meant it or if they were just showing concern as so many of our friends and co-workers had expressed concern over the period of the past couple of weeks.

One of the things that we did was make a list-serve of concerned people so that we could email periodic updates. Depending upon who they were and the personal relationship with Dorene, we would go into more or less detail.

My wife's sister, the one that is a leader in the family, was very helpful during this past trying week. She would come into the hospital most every day. She is intelligent and kind, much kinder than me. She would help me with my charts and the various activities that we needed. My wife was still in pain but we were trying to get her to breath and to walk so that she wouldn't get sicker. The sister helped greatly with all of this. Additionally, she was good company and would take the pressure off of me as I was getting pretty frazzled. Most of all, I could shoot home, hop in the shower, drop of some laundry and come back. Although the breaks were very brief, they gave the chance to get a breath of fresh air and to screw my emotional cap back on. I will forever be indebted to her for her acts of kindness and support.

On many visits, her husband, the nurse would also come. His knowledge about hospitals and medicine was very helpful. It was good to have someone around who could keep me from going off the deep end with worry and anger.

In the same way, my son would come by every night. This would allow me to grab a sandwich and take a break before facing the night, something that I dreaded every day. Sometimes it was just great having him around because my wife would be in better spirits when he was there. After he left, it would be a different story. There were times when I was actually fearful anticipating the long dark nights. I was fearful that she might die and I was fearful that my fear and doubt might show themselves to her.

These moments of lack of confidence or faith, were usually very short. I was determined not to allow myself to be gripped with fear. The fear would remind me that I had to have even greater resolve because my wife was depending upon it. You will experience the same thing, I am sure. You need to stay in the moment, be strong for your loved one, and allow it to pass. Remember, this is about them getting better not about you and your human frailties.

After telling the politicians staff that I didn't need any help, my wife continued to worsen. I had a call into the patients' advocate office because I was not getting any communications. The doctors, as concerned as they were and in spite of my nagging, had not changed their ways. We were treated as if were stupid and all information was kept from us. I was very frustrated. The only one who treated us differently than this was the surgeon but he wasn't around much because he was so busy with surgeries during the day.

That night, as she lay suffering, I told my wife about the call from the local politician. To my surprise, she suggested that I call them back in the morning as she was concerned. This whole situation was a fiasco. She had been there nearly three weeks and had suffered throughout the entire ordeal. The doctors were telling us nothing but something was wrong. They had to put the NG tube back in after my wife had vomited over a gallon of stomach bile all at once (this is not a comfortable thing for a conscious person to experience). We needed all the help that we could get. This was a matter of life and death and it was time to pull out all stops.

In the morning I made the call and within five minutes everything changed. We were immediately getting all sorts of attention. People from the administration showed up. The radiologist came. The head resident showed up and so did the surgeon. From that point on, communications were no longer a problem. Everyone was giving us attention and treating us like intelligent adults.

Dorene wasn't feeling any better at all, she was even sicker and the temperature had returned, but we were getting information. A note to remember here is that you should use any connection that you have to get the attention that your loved one deserves. Believe me, if you don't, they will not get the attention that they deserve and you will always be left in the dark with your questions and thoughts.

That afternoon, someone noticed that the stomach drain, the JP, was filling with green stuff. They sent it to the lab to be analyzed. A CT Scan was ordered. The surgeon showed up and said that his concern was that the green in the bulb looked like bowels so he was trying to find out what went wrong.

Shortly thereafter, the cat was let out of the bag. The surgeon was noticeably shaken. He blamed the radiologists. The radiologist showed up to apologize but pointed out that it was leaking long before they had been involved and, as a matter of fact, he had discovered the leak with the original CT Scan.

Another coincidence happened at this time. My son from Las Vegas, who was very busy trying to get a major project off the ground, had come home to make another visit. My wife always brightens up when her sons are around. She was not feeling well and was scared as she knew something was drastically wrong. Having both sons around her gave her an inner strength that I am certain was instrumental in helping her face the bad news that we were about to receive.

Dorene would need emergency surgery in the morning!

Apparently, when the radiologists thought that they had such an easy time with the wire and the stents, they really hadn't. Instead of putting a stent over the wire and completing the flow of urine from the kidney to the new bladder, they had ripped a hole in the new bladder about an inch wide, severed the ureta from the left side so that it was just floating around the body cavity, and, worst of all punctured a hole in the bowels that was allowing waste to get into her body cavity. There was a fear that this could cause septic poisoning and her kidneys were showing signs of the beginning of failure.

Our surgeon came by and told us what had happened and that he would go back in the morning and reopen the original incision. If he could keep it the same size, he would. He was being accompanied by a world-renown gastro-surgeon in the event that the bowel had been damaged beyond repair and would need some special surgery (colostomy).

His intentions were to go inside her and to start all over again. First he would repair the damage that was done by the radiologists and then he would make sure that everything was done right and fix it.

This, certainly, was a test of our faith. To us, it seemed as if most everything that could possibly go wrong had gone wrong. Everybody in my family disliked the surgeon, at this point, without even knowing him. They hated the hospital and wondered whether or not we had made a drastic mistake going there. Everybody was mad as hell but trying their hardest to remain cool and supportive of Dorene. They knew that they had to remain positive but I could see that there was a lot of whispering going on whenever I returned to the room from stepping out. The bottom line was that everybody was equally scared and mad as hell.

Dorene and I still had confidence in our surgeon. We even liked him. Although, I have to admit, we had tons of doubts. We didn't know who had done what wrong. Honestly, we didn't care at this point. All we wanted was for Dorene to get better. We still had this confidence because of our original research. We had faith that things would improve.

Dorene was too sick to not want to get better. I knew that she was afraid and why shouldn't she be. I put on a brave face, took a deep breath and told her that we were lucky that they had found the mistakes and were going to fix them. Nobody wanted surgery again, as a matter of fact it was something that we had feared from day one, but we knew that we had to face it the next day. I am sure that there were a lot of prayers said that evening by a lot of people, including Dorene and me.

Chapter Five

Emergency Surgery

Early on Saturday, Morning, April 3d, Dorene was slowly transported to surgery. By now all the transportation people knew Dorene and me and were more than happy to go as slow as possible. Even they felt bad for her knowing how much she had suffered. They were aware of the length of her stay and had seen her deteriorate with each trip to wherever they transported her.

The normal pre-op procedures were repeated but this time with less chaos as it was a Saturday morning and there was only one other person in the entire place. Our surgeon was there along with the accompanying surgeons and the assisting residents. They were as reassuring as they could possibly be.

These times of stress will test any religion that you have. Both Dorene and I are pretty steeped in our religion. Honestly, she is more religious than me. At any rate, prior to her going to the hospital, one of her friends had given her a tiny vile of oil that came from some Lebanese saint. Dorene has some Lebanese heritage so the friend thought that this would mean something to her. As a matter of fact, she had rubbed some of it on her incision prior to her first surgery.

I wasn't sure whether this stuff would work or not. But, another big coincidence was that I found it in my gym bag that I had been using to store my dirty laundry at the hospital the very morning of her surgery. Call it superstitious, call it whacky, or just call it an act of faith driven by desperation, but I brought it with me to the pre-op room. I put in on my hand before shaking the surgeon's hand. I managed to put some on my finger and pat the new, hot-shot, surgeon on the back. I put it on Dorene, on the bed, and on the assisting nurse. The bottom line was that I wanted it on everyone and I told Dorene that I did it. She just laughed which was pretty remarkable considering how sick she was and how scared she should have been.

There was a great deal of tension in the room prior to surgery. The surgeons had very serious faces. We were all trying to be jovial and talkative but we all knew that this was a big deal. We remained positive on the exterior but I am certain that we all, including Dorene, had our doubts that we kept to ourselves.

We all told Dorene that we loved her and the nurses wheeled her in for a surgery that we had been told would take about three hours. My sons and I waited in the waiting area.

After about an hour and a half, I saw the hot-shot gastro surgeon leaving the OR and heading home out the front door. I stopped him at the exit and asked him how things went. He told me that everything was under control and that we had a great surgeon who was doing a great job. Then, out the door he went. At least the hospital was pretty consistent in its lack of communications. But, then again, this guy wasn't our doctor and he probably didn't want to say the wrong thing. He gave me the "textbook" reply that he had probably studied and used over and over for many years.

I found this lack of communication to be insulting and arrogant. Any information that you get is very controlled. The nurses have to get so that they really trust you before they dare say anything. It's the hospital's way of controlling anarchy and the law suits that would no-doubt follow.

But they are foolish in this regard. You will gain the information that you want from the nurses and medical staff once you gain their confidence. I think that they almost like giving you the information because they see how frustrated you are and how obnoxiously you are treated by the doctors. The only one who didn't treat us this way was our surgeon but he is a very busy guy and just wasn't around enough.

In about three hours, out came our surgeon. He told us that everything went well. He didn't have to enlarge the original incision. He was able to stitch the rip in the bladder, stitch the hole in the intestine, put stents in properly and reconnect the uretas to the new bladder. He was pleased with the operation and was able to avoid a colostomy. We were all very relieved and cautiously optimistic. You have to be optimistic because it is the only way that you can cling to hope for recovery.

In about an hour I was able to visit Dorene in the recovery room. I told her that everything went well. I also told her that they had used a thinner gauge tube for the NG tube and that she should feel better with it. She was very beat and slept until they got her back to her room.

Her recovery this time around was more like it should have been the first time. She was still nauseous and taking lots of painkilling medications but she was doing better. She still had the nephrostomy tubes in her back diverting the urine but the doctors said that they were going to try to shut them off again in a couple of days and make sure that the urine could come out of the new bladder. Her incision looked good and the JP had the types of post surgery fluids that it was suppose to have without any signs of urine or bowels.

After a couple of days, Dorene couldn't stand the pain from the NG tube anymore and asked for them to remove it. They complied with her wishes and took it out. She vomited once the next day but we figured that was the only price to pay for having the tube taken out a day early and that it was well worth it. She began to get better and was given jello and fluids for the first time in nearly a month.

The nausea never really left her but she was getting better otherwise. When they first shut off the nephrostomy tubes, she was uncomfortable after about an hour. She said that she had a weird feeling in her and asked them to open them up again. This scared us both because we had little confidence in the doctors and knew that they were capable of mistakes and remembered the last problem that we had when they attempted to redirect her urine through her bladder.

Our surgeon devised a plan whereby they would open and shut them over the next few days until her body became accustomed to using the new bladder. He was relatively certain that her discomfort was due to her unfamiliarity with any of this because nothing had worked properly up to now.

He was right! The nurses shut them on and off and I kept records on the grease board. This worked marvelously and in about a week she was using her new bladder, everything was working perfectly and the nephrostomy tubes, although still in place, were completely shut off.

We were very appreciative of the fact that the doctors were keeping us in the loop now. They were telling us their plans and communicating with us throughout the day. I didn't say anything but I thought of how unjust this environment is in this regard. What about all the patients who don't know somebody to stir up the pot? Oh, these doctors, with all of their medical knowledge and skills, could stand to learn so much about communicating with their patients.

The good news was that Dorene was getting ready to go home. She had some problems getting her bowels going as they had been out of order for a month, had holes poked in them inadvertently and been operated on twice. Slowly, and very painfully, I might add, they began working. This was her ticket home.

The surgeon was headed away on vacation for a couple of weeks. By now I had his cell phone number and his email address. He encouraged me to call him or email him. The plan was to get one nephrostomy tube taken out immediately upon his return from vacation and the other a few days later.

He wanted to make sure that everything was working properly with no adverse reactions before removing the tubes that had been put in at such a high price in terms of Dorene's discomfort during the procedure. These tubes could easily be used and reopened in the event that anything was wrong and urine needed to be diverted again.

Our surgeon was a dedicated professional. He genuinely cared about Dorene and was willing to put up with all of my nagging questions. To this day, we are grateful that we chose him even though his team may have made one of the original mistakes by using a stent that was too short and had to be removed. But, then again, perhaps it had just slipped as he had indicated. We didn't really care what it was as he was the guy that always took the time, whenever he was around, to explain in detail what was going on. And, in the end, he was the one who corrected all of the problems.

With that, on April 13th, twenty seven days after her original surgery, my wife was discharged. She was sent home with the tubes in her back but not in use. Her new bladder was working. She was still quite a bit nauseous but happy to be going home. We left without a lot of fanfare, just a wave goodbye to the staff. I think that they were happy for us as they knew that Dorene had suffered more than is normal. More than one person on the medical staff had told us about the importance of getting out of the hospital before you contract some other illness. We were so happy to be headed out.

Chapter Six

Home, Sweet, Home

When Dorene came home from the hospital, she was still sick. She had lost 17 pounds and was weak. She was not eating much, was still nauseous and was in a great deal of pain from the nephrostomy tubes coming out of her back. Plus, she had just endured a couple of major cancer operations and had nearly died from complications.

The tubes were really bothering her. I asked her doctor via email whether or not his partner could remove them. He told me that that he could after one week but first the stents would have to come out. They don't want to remove the tubes until they are very sure that there are no leaks. So, we scheduled the appointment with our surgeon's associate.

The stents came out uneventfully and a couple of days after that the tubes came out. This was a painless procedure that was done in the doctor's office and Dorene immediately started to feel better. Literally, within minutes of the removal of the tubes, she felt the pain subsiding.

This was the best that she had felt in a month. She was still not eating much but the nausea had subsided just a little and she was not in pain. Her first night without the tubes, she slept through the night!

Again, had I not communicated with her surgeon, who was nice enough to encourage me to do so even though he was on a much needed vacation with his family, she would have had to suffer with those tubes for an extra week. You need to be the advocate continually. Her surgeon knew that Dorene had been through plenty and wanted to do anything in his power to help us at this point. We were right about him all along, he really was a good guy.

We went to see her surgeon on the third week after coming home. He gave us the best news ever: Dorene's body was free of cancer. All of the radiology reports had come back negative. She was T-0!

I still remember him telling us this. I actually filled up with tears. What a journey it had been to this point! All of the pain and suffering, both physically and emotionally, had been so that we could hear this result. We were so happy.

Dorene was having some problems with reflux and was sent to a gastroenterologist. He said that her problem was caused by a condition known as gastro paresis which is a slight paralysis of the stomach. This is due, or at least in her case was due, to the length of time that she had spent in the hospital with no food in her system other than the intravenous solutions. He said that it would pass in time and that she should eat small amounts of foods, low in fiber.

As her main caregiver, I became confused by the conflicting reports relative to the nutrition that she needed. On the one hand, we were told before leaving the hospital to give her lots of calories and fiber to get her bowels regulated and now we were being told to give her smaller quantities less in fiber. As part of her aftercare, we asked to see a nutritionist. Again, you must advocate for yourself in these situations.

Armed with our written questions and understandings, we had a consultation with the nutritionist. She put us on the proper diet and told us what foods to eat and not to eat. We found this to be very helpful. The gastroenterologist called every week for the first several weeks. He changed the medicine for the turn for the better.

Once home, there are many things that you can do as a caregiver. These involve the everyday tasks that are normally shared by both parties, keeping a positive vibe at all times, and generally looking after your loved one. You must continue to focus on their well-being and not on yourself.

In the case of my wife, I was aware of the emotional adjustments that she had to make. Her body not only underwent huge trauma, it was also altered in a way that would take time for her to adjust. Presently, she is doing just fine with all of this but I am sure that there are moments when she is troubled. Additionally, the recovery process is long and involved and there are times when she feels better than others. Feeling great, in many cases, is relative to when she was not feeling very well at all, and doesn't mean that she has fully recovered.

I tried to do as many of the mundane tasks around the house as I possibly could for her. You might think that this would create a diversion from one returning to a normal routine. I disagree.

Any task that I could do, first of all, showed that I cared and was vested in her recovery. Secondly, it allowed her to focus on getting better and allowed her to go at her own rate in getting back to doing these things.

When she first came home, I would do everything relative to caring for her. She was still sick. There was daily maintenance to do like washing and disinfecting. There were dressings that needed changing. We had to order supplies and become familiar with the whole process.

In time, as she was feeling better and more familiar with these processes, she started to do them herself. Again, this is a long-time emotional adjustment. But slowly, she did these things and wanted privacy in doing them. I recognized this and gave her all the privacy that she wanted while letting her know that I was available to help in any way if needed.

I made the bed every morning. This isn't a big deal and it is a duty that we both sort of shared prior to the illness. My thinking was that it would be one less thing that she would have to think about and it was an opportunity for me to show her that I care. I, honestly, believe that outward displays of concern and affection are important. It let's your loved one know that you are looking at the physical problem as a problem that will be shared and conquered by the both of you.

My wife needs to take a pill an hour before she eats in the morning and in the evening. I get up a bit earlier than I did before her illness. I go downstairs and make her a cup of ginger tea (she can't have caffeine), make myself a cup of coffee, let the tea steep for 10 minutes and then bring it up to her with her morning medications. Is she capable of doing this? Of course she is but it takes very little effort on my part and the result is that she has one less thing to do in the morning and can rest a bit longer.

Slowly but surely she began to recover. She made the decision to go back to work after a couple of weeks at home. Frankly, she missed being around her friends at the office and didn't care much for being around the house all day. Here, too, we created a routine that still works for us.

After I get dressed in the morning, she hops in the shower and gets ready for work. I go downstairs and prepare her a sandwich for lunch. I make sure that we are always stocked with groceries and that she has plenty of the foods available that she needs. I have a constant list of groceries going. My habit of making lists did not stop with our hospital stay.

The last thing that I do in the morning is make her breakfast. Why do I do this? The answer is simple: I want to make sure that she isn't distracted and that she gets the food that is appropriate for her. She is very capable of doing this. However, how many times have you skipped a meal because you were running late or just didn't feel like doing it? I have many, many, times but with my wife these meal periods are essential to her recovery and I am more than happy to do my share, all the while ensuring that they are done.

All of this may seem like I was smothering her. In some cases, I probably was. However, I let her know at the onset that if I did anything to annoy her that I wanted to know. We all do things that annoy our spouses. I tried my very hardest not to do them. Again, I wanted there to be as little negativity in her life as possible but I knew that she needed to be as positive as possible at all times in order to recover.

For example, I like to fill the waste basket under the sink until it is completely full before taking out the liner, brining it in the garage to the trash can and replacing another liner. My wife, on the other hand, would always take it out in the morning, even if it was only half full, and set it on the kitchen floor to be brought down to the trash on a daily basis. In the past, this would annoy me.

Now, I empty it every single morning whether it needs it or not. It is a very simple thing for me to do and it avoids her finding it under the sink with the resulting sigh of disapproval. We don't need any more sighs of negativity. They create negative energy that usurps the power of healing both physically and emotionally.

The last thing in the world that I want my wife to think about or to be concerned with is all these simple mundane things that crop up in everyday life. There will be plenty of time to give them their proper place after she is healed physically and emotionally. In the meantime, I intend to be as good a person as I can and to relieve her of all these little things. She is under enough stress as it is and she needs to focus on being well.

There is a great deal of emotional stress that comes with having gone through the type of ordeal that she experienced. It takes time to forget it. Perhaps one never does forget. And, there is also the stress of knowing that cancer is a killer and that it can rear its ugly head at any time. We tend to not think about this much when we are healthy but once it has affected you, I believe, there is always a place somewhere in the recesses of your mind where it lingers, just waiting for the right circumstances to come, once again, to the forefront. I don't want to be the cause of any of these unfortunate opportunities.

Another thing that I do is tell her that I love her every, single, time that it comes into my mind. I remember watching her suffer and having those thoughts of just how much I loved her. I remember thinking of the times that I had disappointed her and of the times when I had ignored her. I vowed to myself that this would never be the case again. Life is too precious and my life without her would be empty. So, you can be sure that from now until the end of time, she will never doubt my feelings towards her. I am sure that I will disappoint her again as that is all part of being human. But, you can bet that there will be fewer of these in the future than there have been in the past.

There is a good lesson here for us all to learn. Don't wait until it's too late to develop this understanding. In life, we are all so busy. We take for granted the things around us that mean the most to us. That is, until we fear losing them. And then, we are reminded of their importance.

If you are aware, you can use your loved one's illness to refocus on those things that are important. The comfort and sense of being in the right place that comes with this recognition is a huge benefit to both the sick person and to those around him or her. Don't wish that you had said or done something different. Just do it and you will see how good it allows you to feel.

Chapter Seven

Man-up: It's not about you

Please pardon the reference to gender. It is not meant to be a sexist remark and I apologize if it comes across as such. What I mean by this is that regardless of your sex, there will be many times throughout your loved ones crisis that there will be a need for you to forget about your troubles and focus on those of your sick loved one. You have to "bite the bullet" and forget about your troubles and focus on the ill person.

When someone is seriously ill in the family, everyone is affected. Everyone feels troubled. Everyone is concerned.

Sometimes, your concern will make you feel bad for yourself. This can happen at the most unexpected time. It may just start with a sort of depressed feeling but it will almost always end with some outward display.

You may find yourself telling someone about the details of your loved one's illness. I am convinced that when we do this, we are looking for sympathy. You may not be doing it overtly, but somehow or another, you are really looking for some sympathy and some sort of validation of all that you have been going through.

There are other times when you just really feel bad for yourself. You are sitting on a big, old, pity pot and are in a funk. Woe is me. How could this be happening to me? My life is upside down. It will never be the same. I am miserable, etc., etc.

The more you think this way, the more you will have negative thoughts. A better way of handling this is to be aware that you will have these thoughts and to expect them. Then, when they come, just say hogwash! Quit feeling bad for yourself and remember that it is not about you but about your loved one getting better. You can't afford to let down your guard.

All of this sounds pretty elementary. It is not. You need to be constantly aware of your negative feelings. Be on guard! Don't allow a "mountain to be made out of a mole hill." The only mountain that you have to worry about is that of helping your loved one back to a full recovery, emotionally, spiritually, and physically.

Whenever your problems seem overwhelming, just take a look around. I bet that you can find plenty of other people who have problems that make yours look minor in comparison. I, personally, think that this awareness and perspective is a good defense.

When I think about all of our awful experiences, I am reminded that, in the end, my wife was made better. Perhaps she has had to endure far more than was originally planned, but the medical world is not perfect. They, like you, make mistakes. The mistakes, in my opinion, should not be the area of focus. Your focus, and that of your sick loved one, has absolutely got to be on the challenges of the present.

I am a pretty independent guy and tend to handle my own problems. However, this experience has taught me that you should take all the help that you need. Remember, there are other people who feel quite bad for all that your loved one has and will continue to endure. If they offer to help, and if you need the help, don't be stubborn. This is no time to be a martyr, let them help as it will be therapeutic to them as well.

There is a huge difference between accepting the generous offerings of others and in feeling badly for yourself. I don't think that this acceptance should be construed, in any way, as a weakness or a succumbing to feelings of self doubt.

My wife is very close to her boss. He is a bright, decent man. Throughout this entire ordeal, I would text him and he would do the same to me, about 10 times a day. I now realize just how therapeutic this was for me. I hope that it was for him as well. I guarantee you that it made me feel better knowing how much he cared. Far more importantly, Dorene appreciated his condern.

In the case of my wife, the daily visits from the visiting nurse once we were home were very therapeutic. Not only was her medical advice and experience beneficial, but just the fact that Dorene had another person to talk to about her concerns and doubts proved very helpful. As a matter of fact, my wife became dear friends with her nurse and now sees her often socially even though the visits stopped weeks ago.

I just think that any energy that you waste by allowing negative thoughts to affect you is exactly that, wasted energy. And frankly, you won't have any energy to waste. You need all of it to remain positive and to beat off the demons that seem to want to tug at you and bring you down.

Somewhere, someplace, I once read that if you can't make it, you should fake it. There is a lot to be said for this. If you are feeling gloomy, try looking in the mirror and smiling. I bet that you will start to feel better. If you're consumed with troubling thoughts, shake them off. Get out of yourself and interact with others on entirely different matters. In a short period of time you will probably start to feel better.

I have always had the good fortune of enjoying my work. But after my return to work, it took on a whole new light. My professional life was a source of a return to normalcy for me. The routines and the normal interactions that I had always enjoyed but taken for granted were a source of real pleasure. You see, in spite of your earth shattering dilemma, life goes on. Live every bit of it when you are not dealing with your sick loved one and you will find that it helps you get through the tough spots.

If you feel yourself going to a place that you don't want to be emotionally, remember your job. You are an advocate, a caregiver, a devoted partner, and a vested component in your loved one's recovery. These roles require certain responsibilities. One of them is to remain positive and not to allow negative thoughts and gloom to affect your behavior. If you remain cognizant of this, I suspect that you will do just fine. If you can't, get the help that you need.

Again, this is just my personal story. I recognize that I am not a mental health genius and that there are plenty of professional folks who would probably say that my advice is something less than text book. However, I also bet that they probably can see where I am coming from and have lots of theories that would say about the same thing in an entirely different way.

We are all different. We come from different backgrounds and live in different environments. But, if cut, we all bleed. Emotionally, this is the way that I have dealt with this ordeal and it has worked for me. I hope that it will work for you as well.

Get over your own individual problems and inconveniences that are created by your loved one illness. It's not about you: it's about helping your loved one recover!

Chapter Eight

To Sue or Not to Sue

Every time that I tell a close friend about our ordeal, they end up asking if I am going to sue the hospital or the doctors. I don't have any specific answers for you relative to this subject but I think it might be worthwhile to share my thoughts on the subject.

My entire life, I have advocated for the small business person. I have seen them make plenty of mistakes and pay the price. I have also seen them lose fortunes as they have been victimized by people and legal professionals who are looking for nothing but financial gain. In my role as an advocate for these small business people, I have come to think less of people who seek damages just because they can get them rather than because of any deliberate and malicious wrong doing on the part of the small business person.

For this reason, I never once thought about suing the doctors or professionals who made mistakes and caused my wife to suffer far more than was necessary. All of these people wanted to help my wife. Things just went bad. Without exception, they all cared for her and hoped that they could make her better. They were all good men and women trying their best to help her. They were compassionate and tried to be reassuring.

My anger during the process was more at the system than at any one person. The medical world has this "code of silence" whereby the doctors keep their opinions to themselves. The nurses are way down the food chain in terms of the hierarchy that exists. Their opinions may be relevant behind closed doors, although I doubt it seriously, but they are not allowed to voice them to the person who needs to know the most, the patient.

I think the doctors and hospitals are afraid of being sued so they clam-up and don't offer any more information than that which you can drag out of them. I was disturbed by this and most of my anger and criticism was due to it.

However, the doctors, radiologists and nurses are all good people. They really do care. Why else would they be so dedicated and give up so much to pursue this profession that consumes so much of their lives?

Now I don't know about you, but I have made plenty of mistakes in my job. As a matter of fact, I sort of believe that if you don't make a mistake or two along the way, you probably aren't trying hard enough. How could I sue these good people because they made a mistake or two? I wish that they hadn't and I wish that my wife had not suffered as much as she did, but none of it was intentional. Whether it had to do with incompetence or not, I will never know. I just hope that there were lessons learned so that some other poor soul will not have to experience the unnecessary suffering that my wife did.

I know enough about law, insurance companies and the court to that if we were to sue we would probably get some money. We could get a good law firm to take our case on a contingency basis and let them go to town. They could file papers, name names, and create a whole lot of worry. Whether or not it would ever go to trial would probably only be dependent upon what they were seeking in damages. I bet the insurance company or companies, depending up how far they spread their web, would end up settling for a sum of money.

But, would this money do anything to help my wife get better? Would it do anything to alleviate the pain that she had endured? In our case the answer is an emphatic no.

I will say, however, had my wife suffered a prolonged or permanent damage due to the mistakes that were made, I would reconsider all of this. But the answer to this is that, fortunately, her problems began to end with the emergency surgery when they were able to repair all of the wounds that they had caused along the way.

In fact, when we began this journey, my wife's life was threatened by a vicious cancer that was invasive and aggressive. We left that hospital with no cancer in her body. She was bloodied, battered and torn but the original goal of getting rid of this demon had been met. So, I decided not to sue anyone and to keep it out of my mind. After all, I needed to stay positive and what could be more negative than thinking of accusations, lawyers and depositions. No thanks, I didn't want to relive any of this and I didn't want any "blood money" and was very grateful that they had removed the immediate threat to her life: cancer.

However, there was one thing that bothered me to no end.

When we were in the hospital, we managed to secure a private room. I knew that the fee for this was an additional $150 per day and that my health insurance would not cover this expense. Fortunately, this was not a lot of money to me and was very affordable. As I mentioned earlier, if you can get a private room and can handle the expense, make sure that you do. It is worth every penny that it will cost you.

About a month after returning home, I finally received the bill from the hospital for the balance do for the private room. It was roughly

$3500, an amount that I could very easily pay. However, it just didn't set well with me.

I am a principled guy and I have literally grown up in the restaurant business. In our business, it's all about taking care of the guest. You want them to have a good experience so that they will tell others and so that they will return. Attracting new customers is important, but making sure that those that you have are satisfied is really what you try to do on a daily basis. All good restaurateurs try to exceed the expectations of their customers.

This bill was for roughly 24 days in a private room. The entire process was to take 7-10 days. Due to my wife's strong physical condition, most of the doctors thought that her stay would be about a week.

I was aggravated to think that the hospital, whose care my wife was under, had made mistakes that had nearly cost her life and had created great suffering. And now they were charging me this fee for this prolonged period that they had caused. I was so angry that I didn't tell my wife and decided that I should do nothing for a couple of days until I had time to process it all. The reason I didn't tell my wife was because I was feeling pretty negative and I didn't want it to rub off on her. She had enough to deal with just trying to recover.

Finally, it was a Friday morning when I called the woman who had given me her business card the day that I had involved the local politician with the hospital administration. I left her a message and she called me back within the hour. I told her that I was upset and wanted to see the President of the hospital. I wanted the chance to look him in the eye and to let him explain to me why I should pay this bill.

I told her that I was not threatening but that my wife had endured too much pain after we met last for me to pay this bill. I told her that I came from a background in which you "comp" a meal if the customer justifiably complains about the poor service or quality.

She asked me to explain because she was unaware of any of the problems that had taken place after the day that we originally met. I slowly and methodically explained much of what you have read. At the end of it all, she said that it would not be necessary for me to come in and that she would explain all of this to the President of the hospital and would get back to me at the beginning of the week.

On the following Monday morning, she called me and told me that the case had been reviewed and that everybody involved agreed that I would not have any additional charges and the balance on my account would be zeroed out! This made me feel good. It, honestly, wasn't about the money as much as it was about the principle that I felt like we were being treated poorly.

In a hospital setting, there are many different departments. Billing and accounts receivable have nothing to do with patient care. They are understandably clueless about it. One hand has no clue what the other hand is doing.

In this particular case, I was advocating one more time. I hope that I was advocating, not only for my wife and for me, but for everybody in the hospital. If you are unhappy, you have to let them know. Don't sit idly by an allow wrongdoings to take place. Not only will it cost you money, it will fill you with negativity and that can come with a far greater cost to you and the person you are trying to help recover.

I bet that there is nobody connected with the hospital or the doctors that gives a hoot about your emotional level. You're the advocate, not the patient. They probably don't even buy into my theory relative to remaining positive and not allowing negativity to come creeping in. But they are so wrong.

You see, in my opinion, when you are out of their sight or responsibility, it's over for them. I am sure that they hope you recover but for the vast majority of them you are just a distant memory. There are lots more patients to treat.

At one point doing our stay the Beth, Israel, Deaconess Hospital in Boston, I thought of just leaving and getting Dorene to another hospital. I could look out her window and see Dana Farber. But a medical friend advised me against doing this. He said that if I did, the team could care less. They would just move on to the next patient and I would be on my own with a new team who wouldn't take any ownership in the problem. He thought that I was better off staying for this reason.

The bottom line is that your emotional state is important to your loved one's recovery. Try to stay as positive as possible. To me, lawyers, dispositions and accusations are counterproductive to healing. I wanted no part of it.

Chapter Nine

Conclusion

I hope that this book will help you and your loved one get better. All of the experiences that I have shared are real. There is no fiction in it. As I mentioned in the preface, my only goal is to help others.

At times it may seem as if I am trying to change the hospitals and the medical system. Although I would like to achieve this, it would take much more than my observations to do so. I do hope, however, that some medical professionals somewhere will read these passages and think about the way that they communicate with their concerned patients. Wouldn't it be nice if nobody had to use the clout of a local politician to get the information that they deserve?

My wife is doing very well. She is four moths post surgery and has returned to work. She still tires more easily than prior to her ordeal but is gaining strength on a daily basis. Each week she looks and feels better than she did the week before.

She has not returned to the gym, nor have I. She walks about three miles a day and I accompany her when I can. Emotionally, she is doing fine. She had a lot of adjustments to make and is making them. The things that we thought were pretty awful at the beginning have found their proper place in terms of their relevance.

I haven't returned to the gym because I don't want to remind her of any limitations that she now has due to her surgery. Instead, we are having our basement done over and will turn it into a gym that will allow us both to enjoy working out together.

Our relationship remains strong. We tell each other that we love one another every, single day. We are grateful to the medical professionals that saved my wife's life and have told them so.

The many cards and flowers that we received during my wife's illness taught me another lesson. If you learn of someone who is sick or who has suffered a loss, don't think about reaching out to them, just do it. Those cards and flowers meant a great deal to Dorene and me during her illness and recovery. I hope that ours will to our friends when they find themselves in similar situations. I know that yours will when you send them to your friends, as well.

The little things in life that bothered me greatly, in the past, seem to have found a better place on my list of priorities. They are way down at the bottom where they belong. When I find myself turning negative or letting little things get to me, I try to put them in their proper place.

Spiritually, both Dorene and I remain strong in our faith. I choose to believe that all of those coincidences that we experienced were answers to prayers and kind thoughts of many, many, people who care about us both. I suspect that if you allow yourself to see them, you will realize that these same "coincidences" are happening in your life as well.

I have always had a tendency of waiting to really appreciate things until there was a threat that I might lose them. I have no idea why this is so but suspect it is human nature.

This situation and experience has allowed me and my wife to refocus. We enjoy life, our families, our friends, our jobs and each other. This appreciation is a gift that has come from all that we endured. Nothing will ever change this as long as we live.

You are taking on a very important role whether you wanted it or not in becoming the caregiver for your loved one. It involves the spiritual, the emotional and the physical. Remain positive, stay in the present, be an advocate and learn all that you can about your loved one's problem. I am sure that you will do just fine as long as you remember: It's not about you: it's about your loved one getting better!

This book has been written from my perspective: that is, one of a caregiver. Believe me when I tell you that my experience paled in comparison to those of my wife who had to endure the physical pain. I am keenly aware of her sacrifice and suffering. I witnessed almost every minute of it.

My research has not ended. I am still reading and writing things down on paper. I know that the surgeon removed the cancer from my wife's body but am still concerned that this tumor may have been the symptom of a malady that exists that allowed it to grow.

I am on shaky ground on this particular point, but I have friends who have experienced similar things and have focused on diet and nutrition to change their bodies' chemistry and are doing great now. We are looking into this and are contemplating a diet based on plant foods rather than animal foods.

We will have a lot of research to do before I feel confident enough to talk in detail about it. However, it makes sense to us and I can't see where it can do anything other than help us both. So, I believe that a change in diet is probably the next step for us.

In no particular order, I will leave you with a brief summary of things that I learned as a caregiver that will help you, I am sure:

1) Stay in the Present—just deal with what is and don't wander off into a future that may never happen the way that you fear.

2) Show demonstrative affection to your loved one—you know that you already feel this way. There is no sense in keeping it a secret now.

3) Learn as much as you can about your loved one's illness—knowledge will help you to understand things that will be presented to you and empower you in making all sorts of decisions.

4) Be an advocate continually—this is your primary function. Whether in a hospital or at home, you are the advocate. Nobody cares more about your loved one than you. Be assertive when necessary.

5) Write everything down—questions, facts, observations. Your writings will prove helpful to the medical people but, most of all, your loved one will benefit greatly, in so many different ways.

6) Fear is the opposite of faith and to the extent that you have one, you will not have the other. Find faith in something whether it's a spiritual faith, one created by knowledge, or one based on the confidence you have in others.

7) Put the needs of your loved one above your own—respect their wishes. It's all about them, not you. You've got plenty of time to get all the attention that you need, focus on your sick loved one.

8) Focus on the symptoms, not the blame. If your finger is bleeding it doesn't matter how it was cut. All that matters is that you stop the bleeding. There will be plenty of time after the crisis has passed to focus on the underlying causes.

9) Remain positive—don't allow gloom or fear to bring you to a place that won't help you or your loved one. If you need help, get it, But, if you focus on the sick person and not yourself, you will be able to remain positive.

10) If hospitalization is required, try to get a private room if you can possibly afford one.

11) Use every connection that you have or skill that you possess to gather information. Befriend the nurses and the staff, use connections, ask for a patient advocate, stop at nothing. You are an intelligent person and need to know what is happening.

12) Accept the help of others. There are lots of people that care about your loved one and want to help. Let them! It may help you garner the strength that you need to be a better advocate.

God Bless you and your loved one!

www.ingramcontent.com/pod-product-compliance
Lightning Source LLC
Chambersburg PA
CBHW022133170526
45157CB00004B/1868